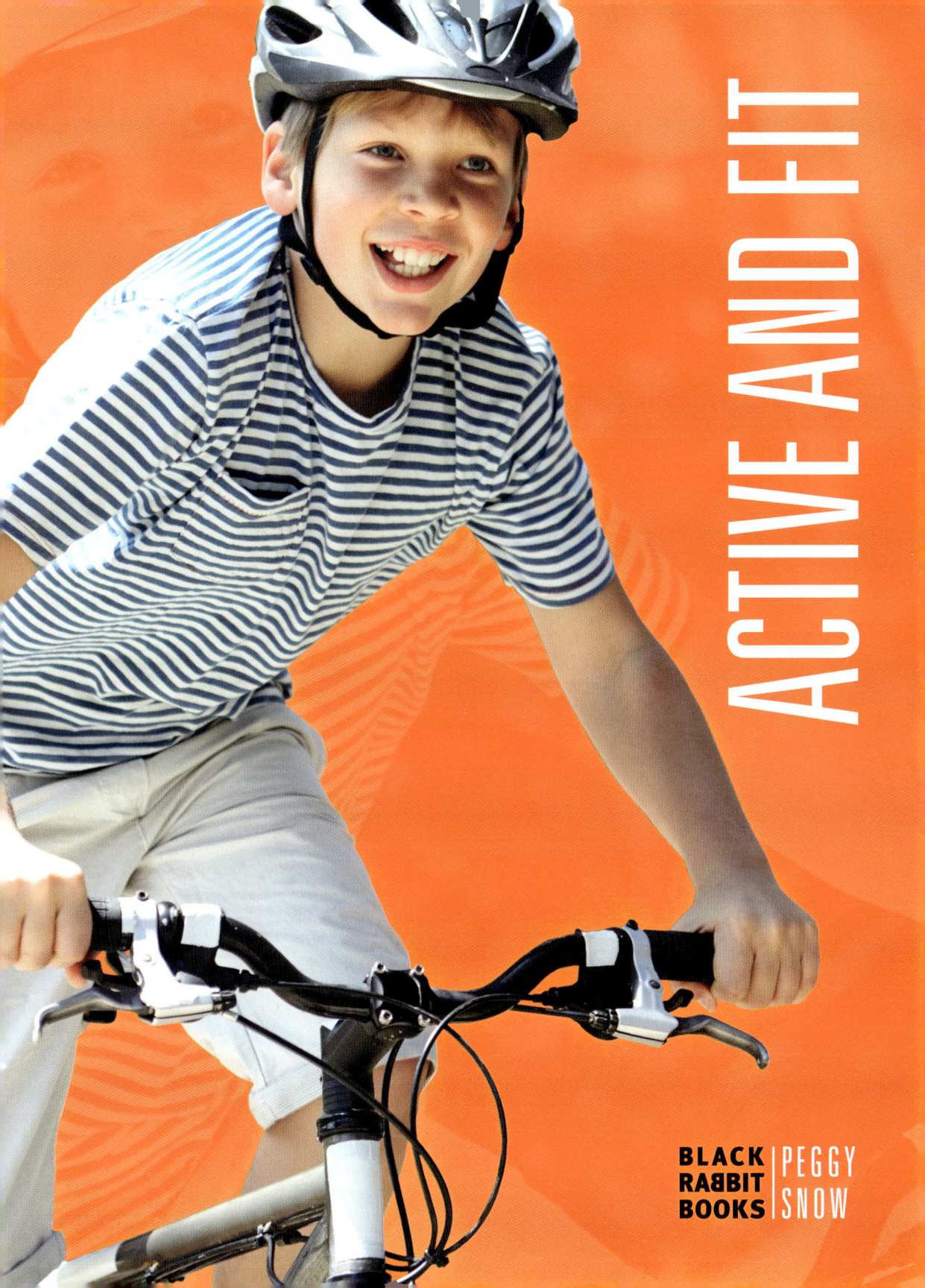

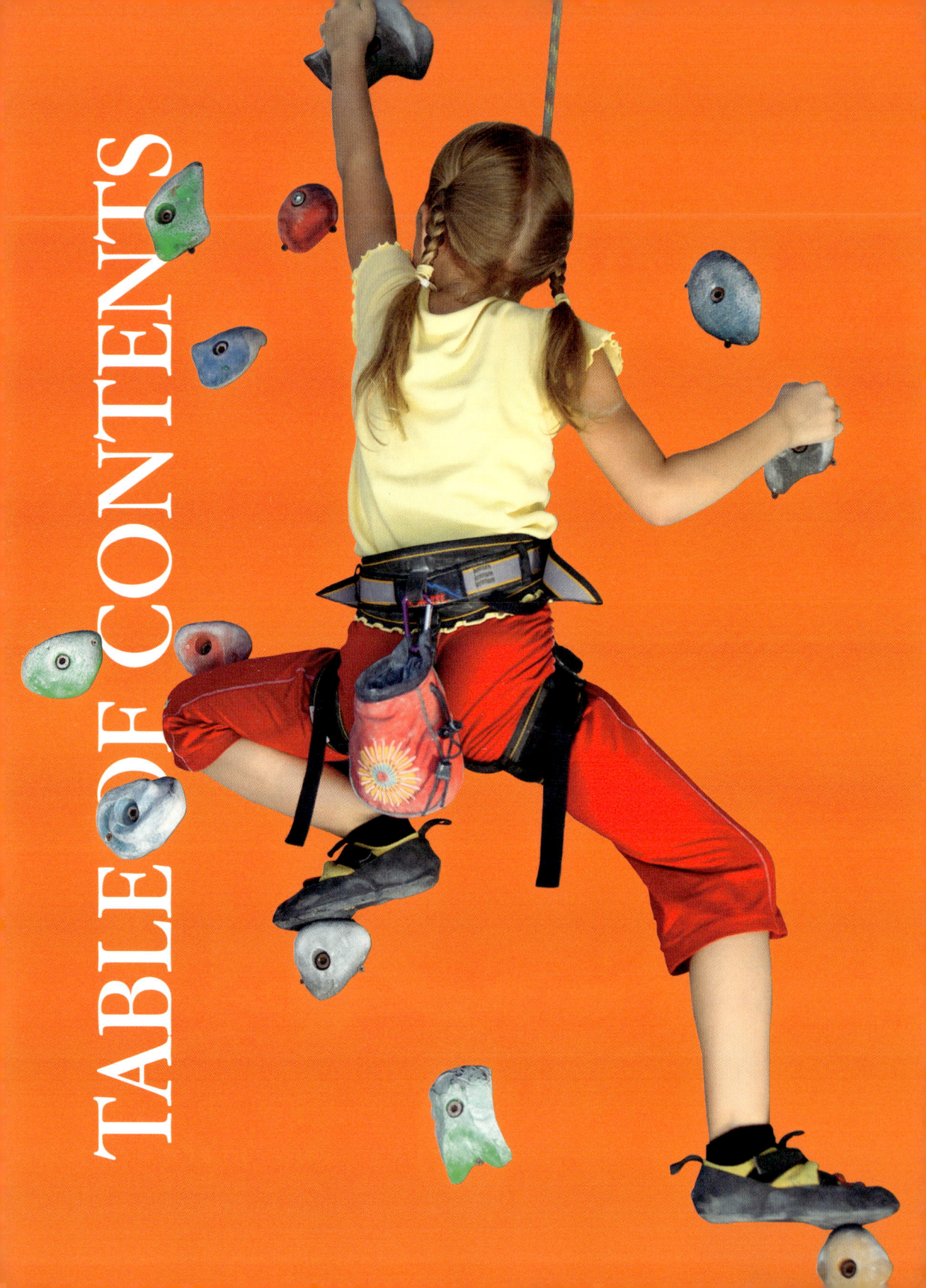

TABLE OF CONTENTS

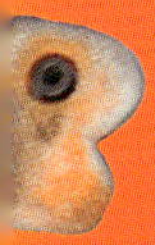

1. Being Active Is Awesome 4

2. Being Active Is Smart 6

3. Muscle Builders 10

4. Heart Helpers 13

5. Get Bendy 16

6. Have Fun with Fitness 19

More to Explore 22

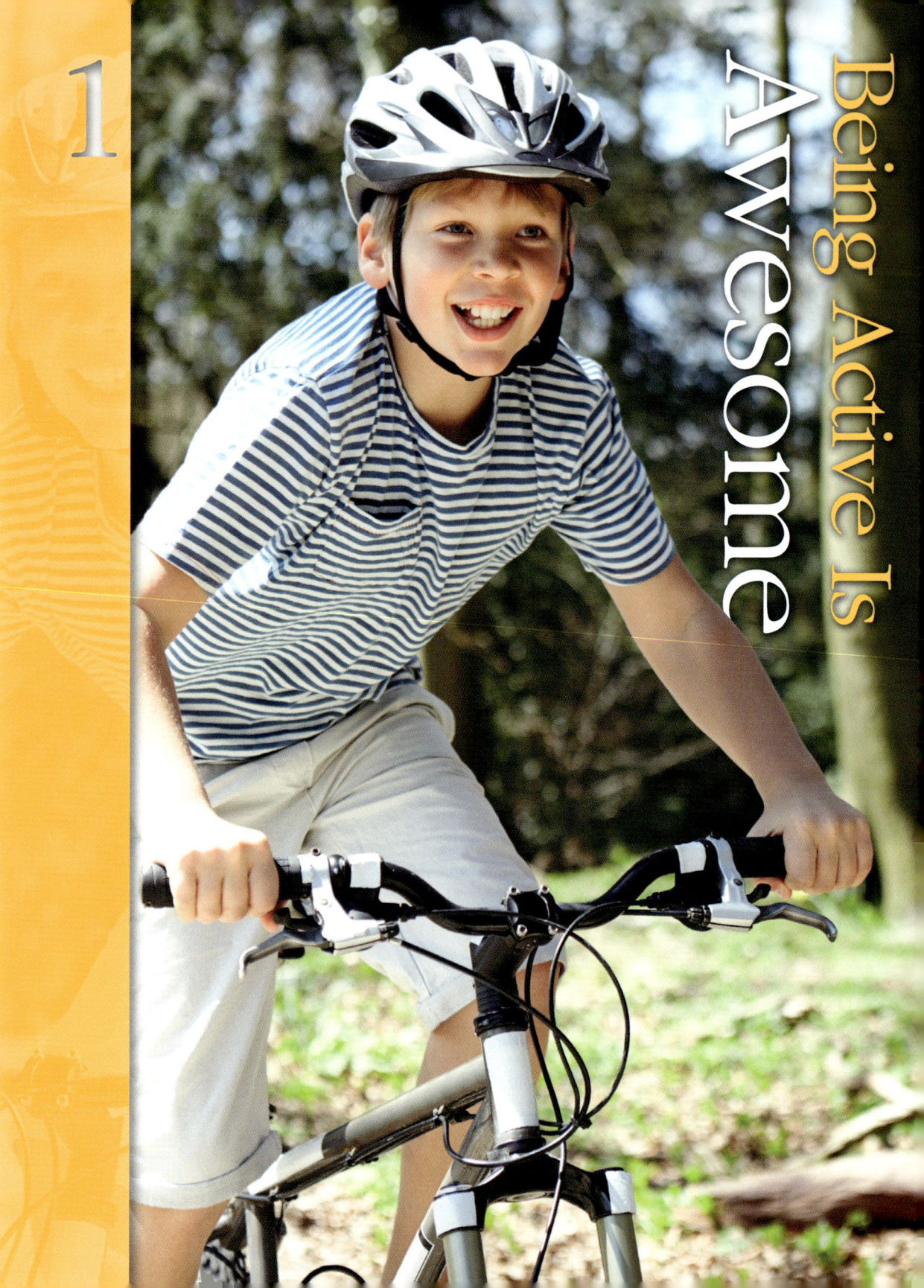

1

Being Active Is Awesome

When you're active, you get fit. When you're fit, you feel good. You're healthy and strong. You have more energy. Your body weight is right for you.

What are ways to be active? You can run, jump, dance, and climb. Do push-ups and crunches. Ride a bike. Touch your toes.

Being active builds endurance. You are stronger and more flexible. You can play longer and move more. Can you be active for an hour a day?

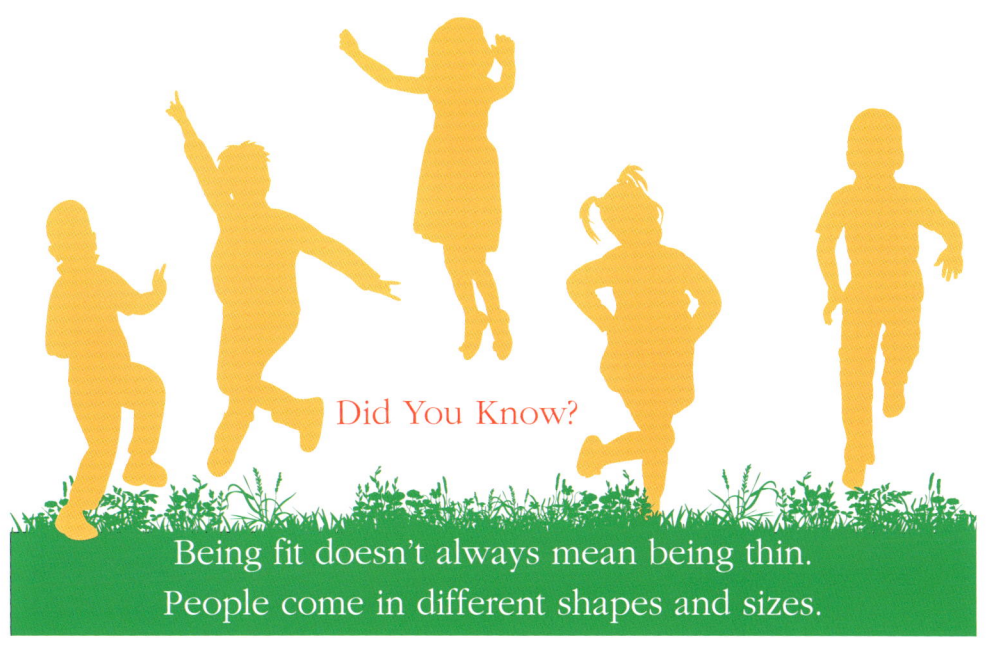

Did You Know?

Being fit doesn't always mean being thin. People come in different shapes and sizes.

Being Active Is Smart

2

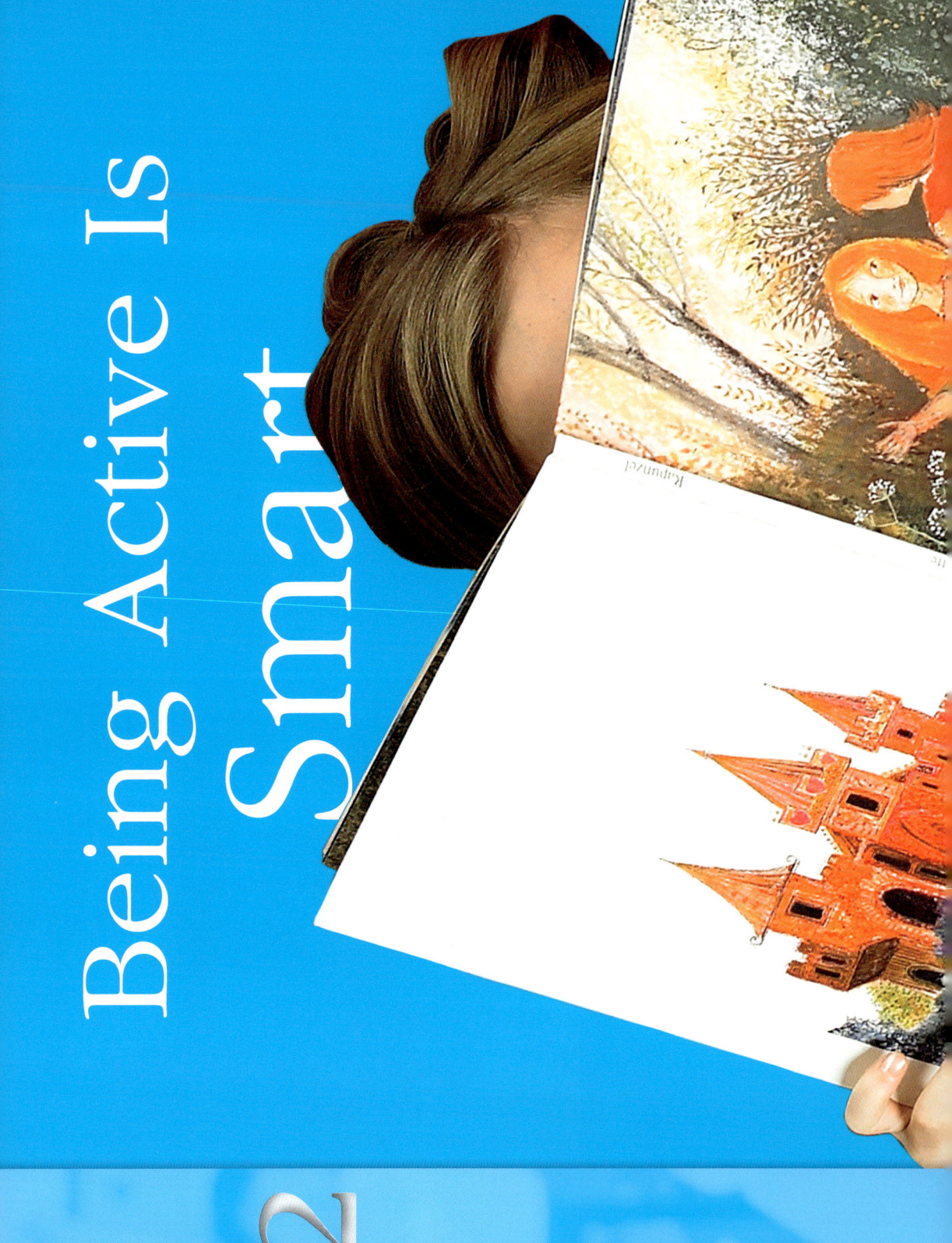

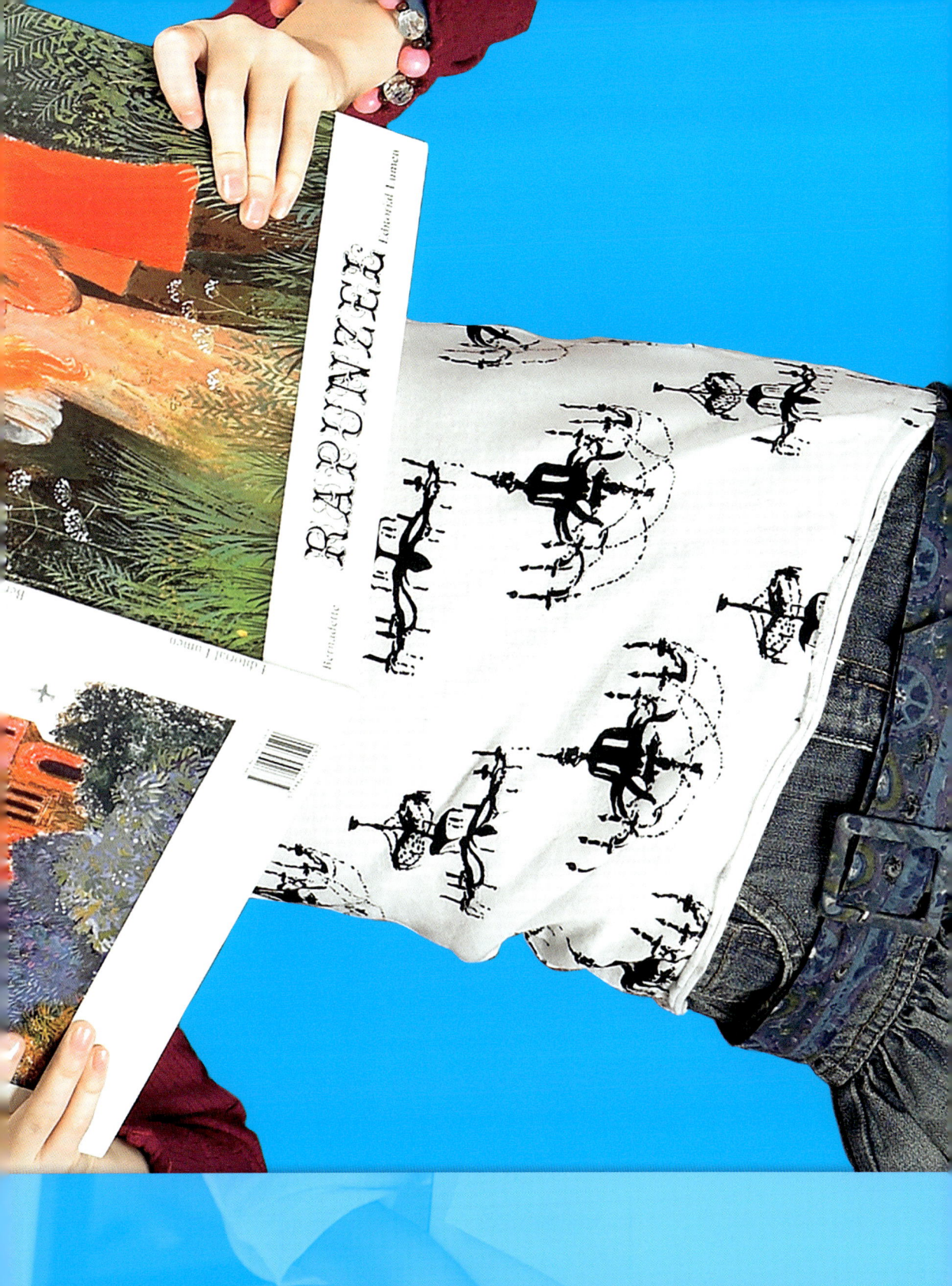

Being active is good for your body. It's also good for your brain. Special chemicals in your brain notice when you're active. They get more active too. They give you more energy. They make it easier to focus and concentrate. You're in a better mood.

Guess what? When you're active and fit, you're more ready to learn. You do better in school. Plus, learning is more fun. Being active even helps you sleep better at night.

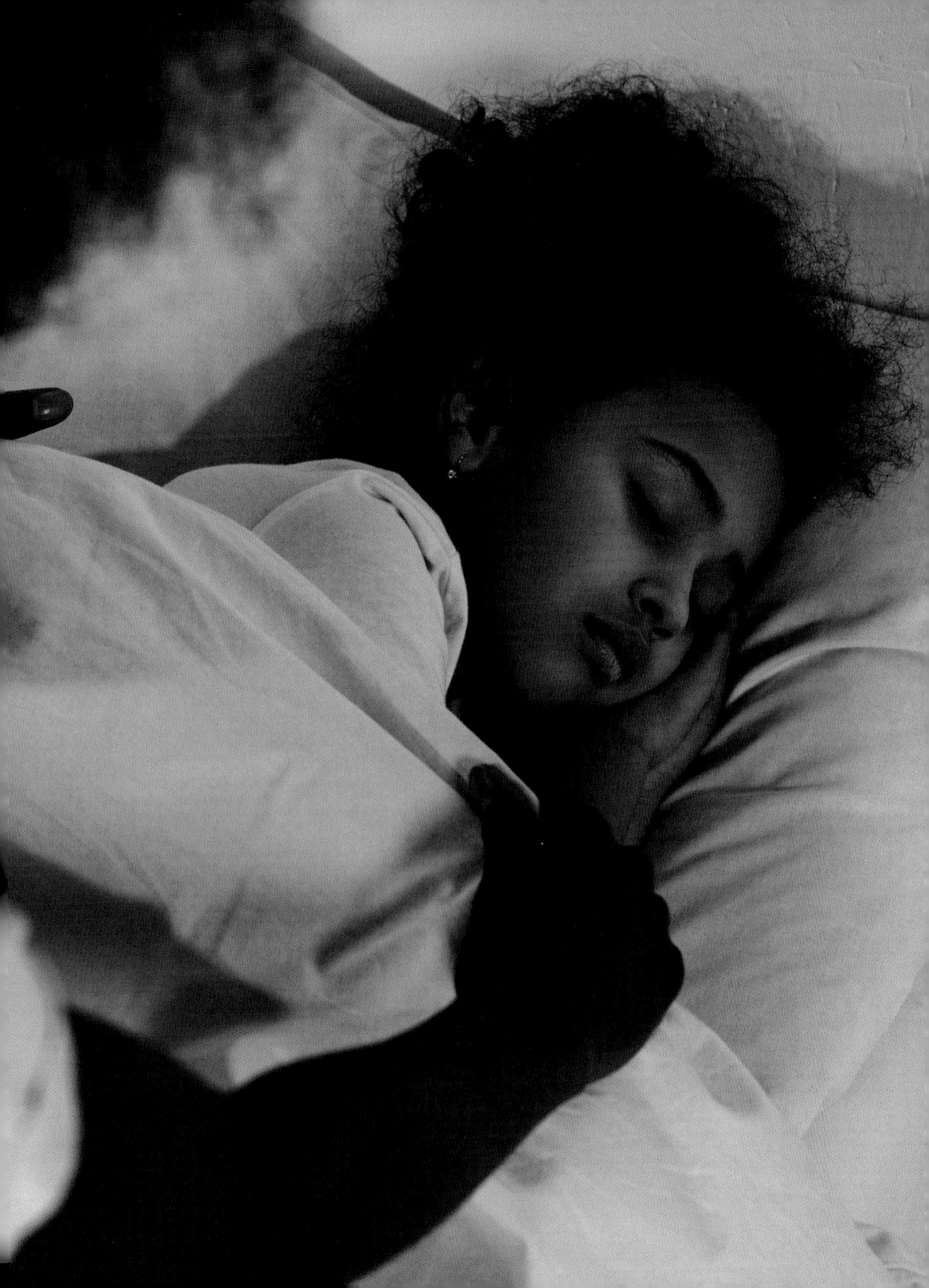

Muscle Builders

3

10

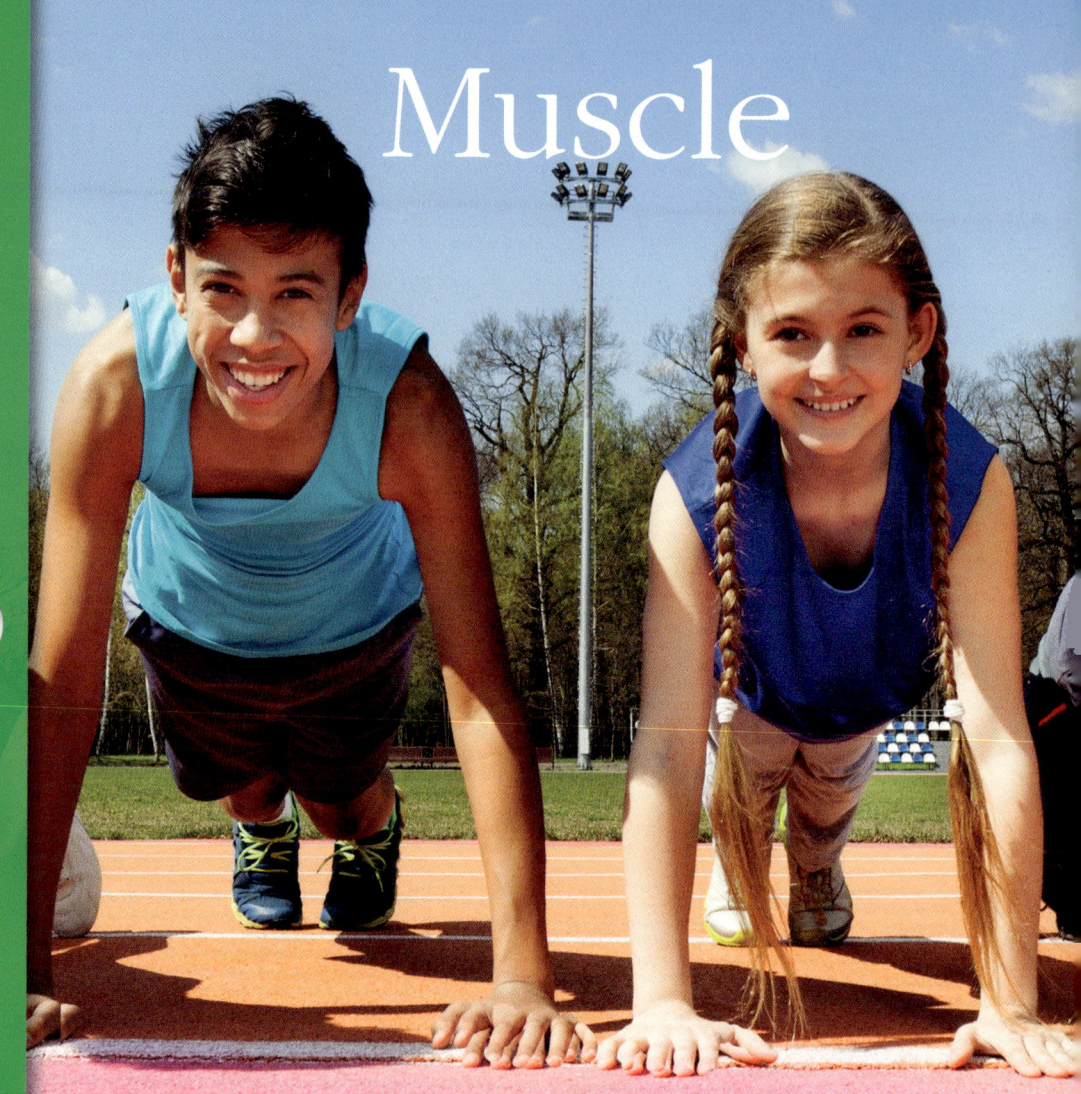

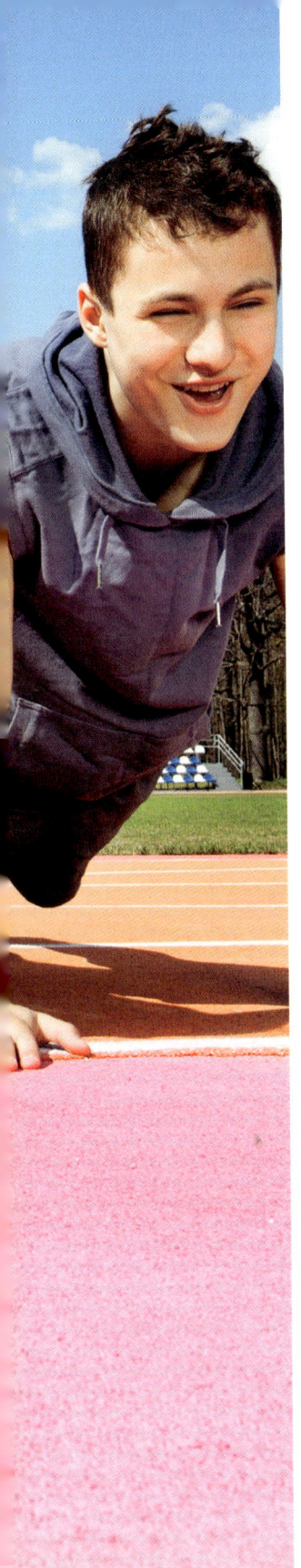

Just moving your body makes it stronger. When you run, skip, and jump, your body builds muscle.

Strong muscles help improve your **performance**. You get better at things like soccer, skating, and dancing.

How else can you build muscle? You don't need to lift weights. Try push-ups or sit-ups. These build your **core muscles**. Or climb the monkey bars or jungle gym. These will build your arm and leg muscles.

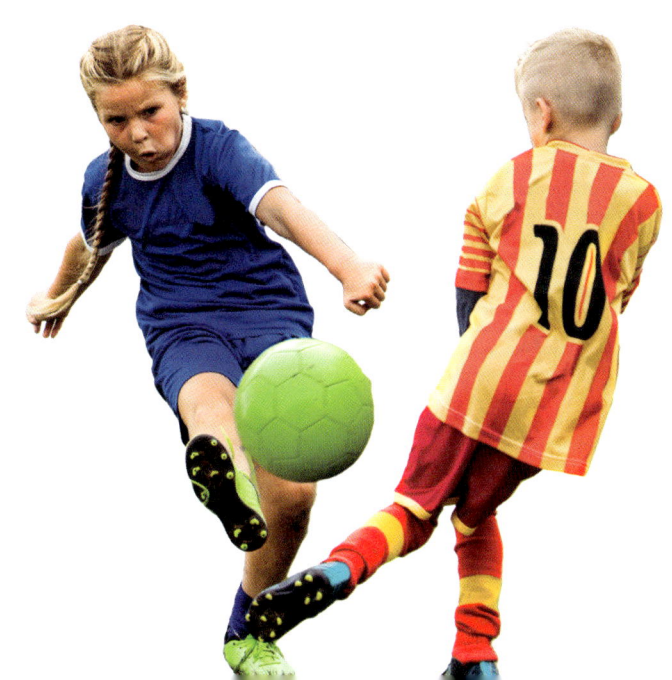

Did You Know?

Would you like big muscles, like a pro athlete? You'll have to wait until **puberty** for that. But you can build strong, healthy muscles now.

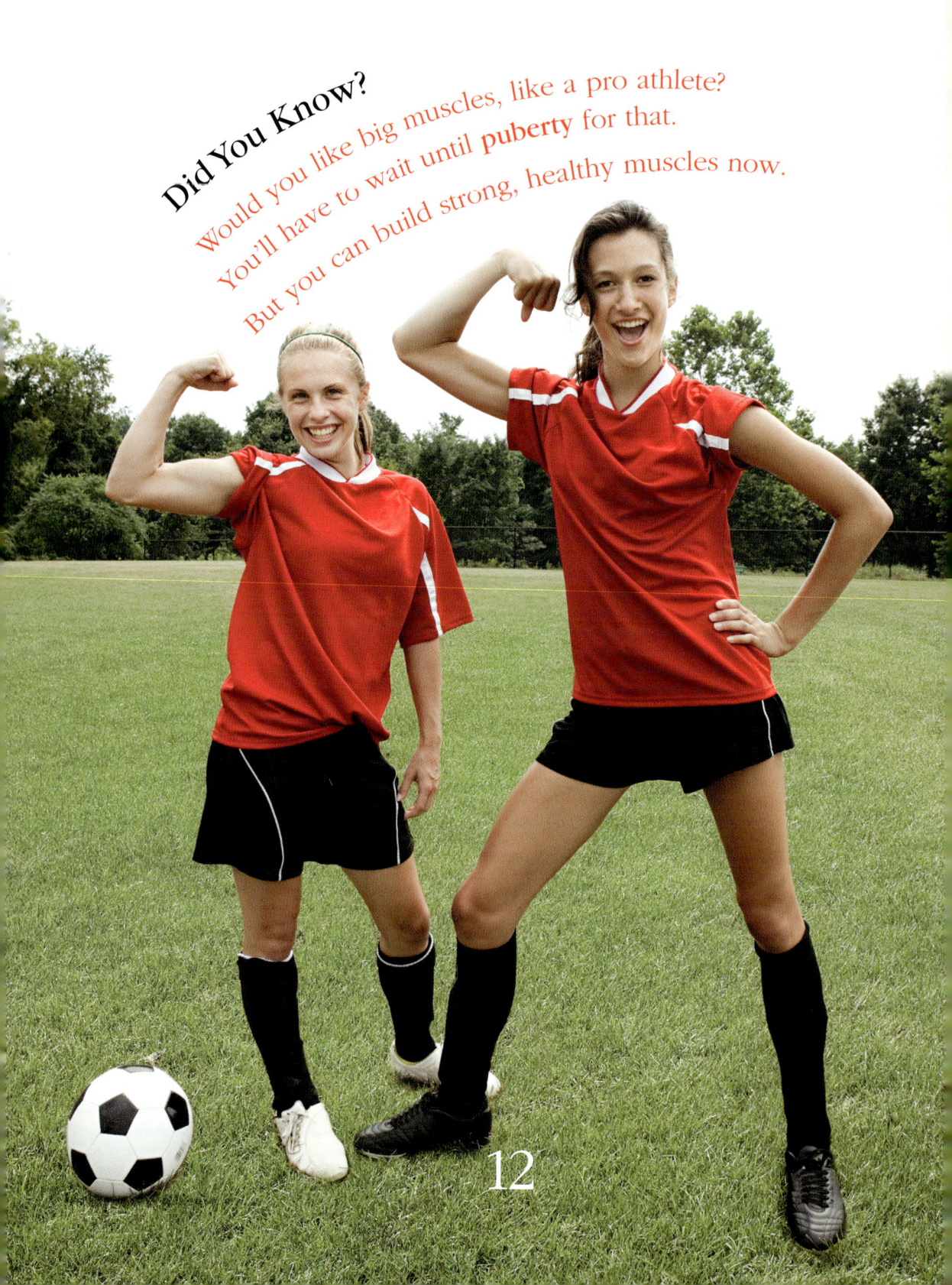

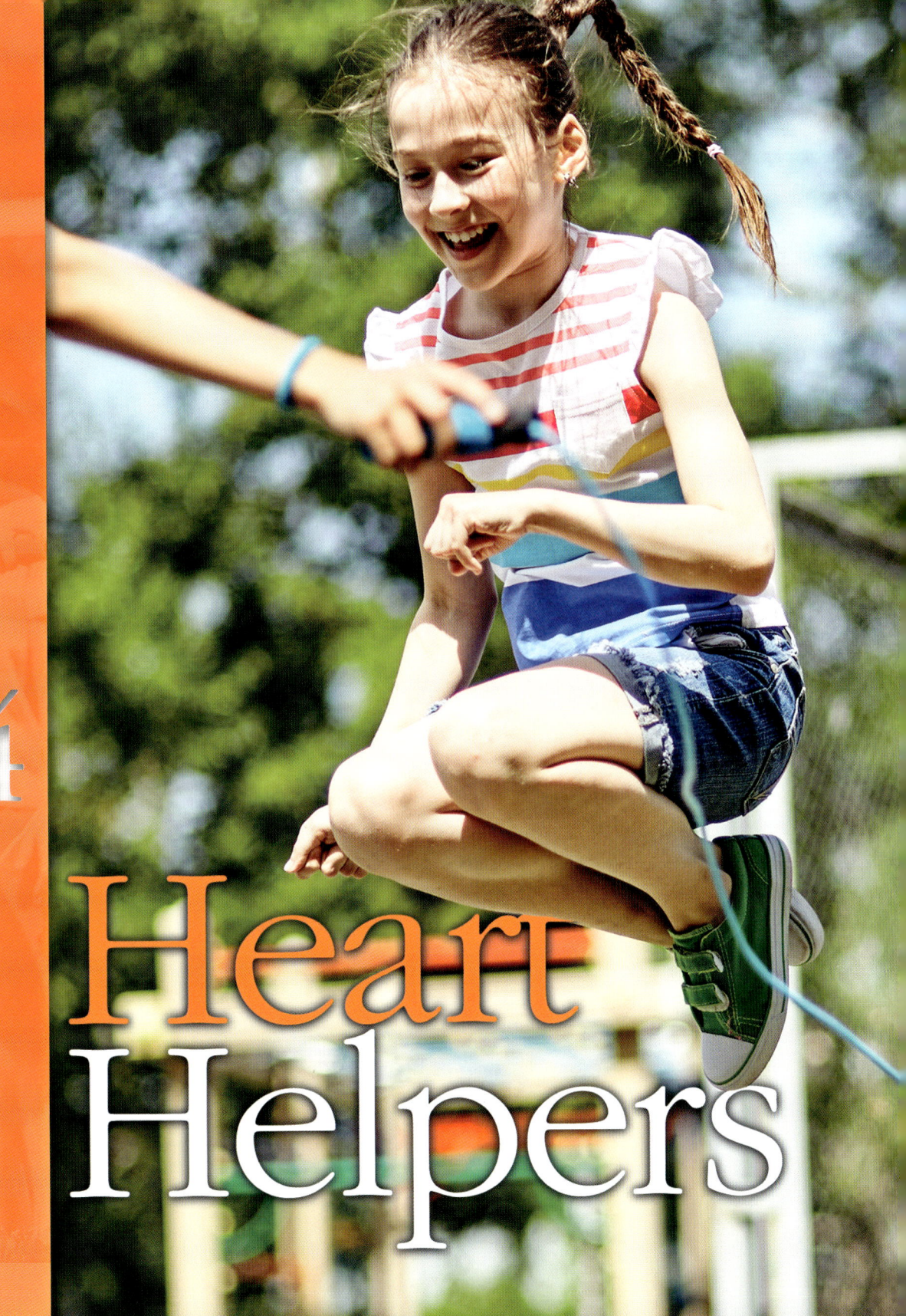

4

Heart Helpers

Your heart is your most important muscle. Being active makes your heart happy.

When you run, bike, and jump rope, your heart beats harder. Your breathing speeds up. More oxygen goes to your heart. Then it gets pumped out to the rest of your body.

When your heart is strong, you don't tire as easily. You can play sports and activities longer.

If you sweat, that's okay. Sweat is your body trying to cool down.

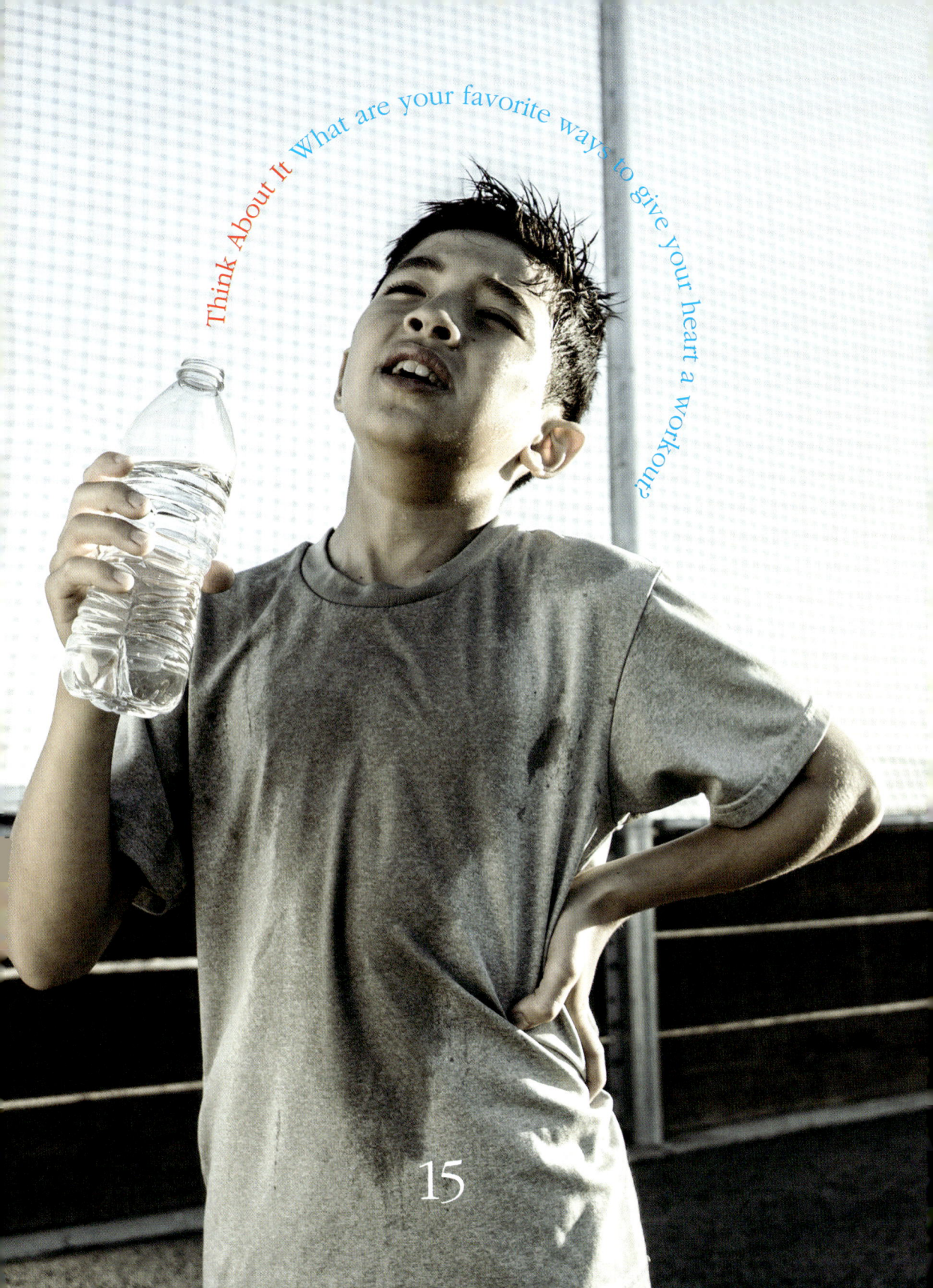
Think About It What are your favorite ways to give your heart a workout?

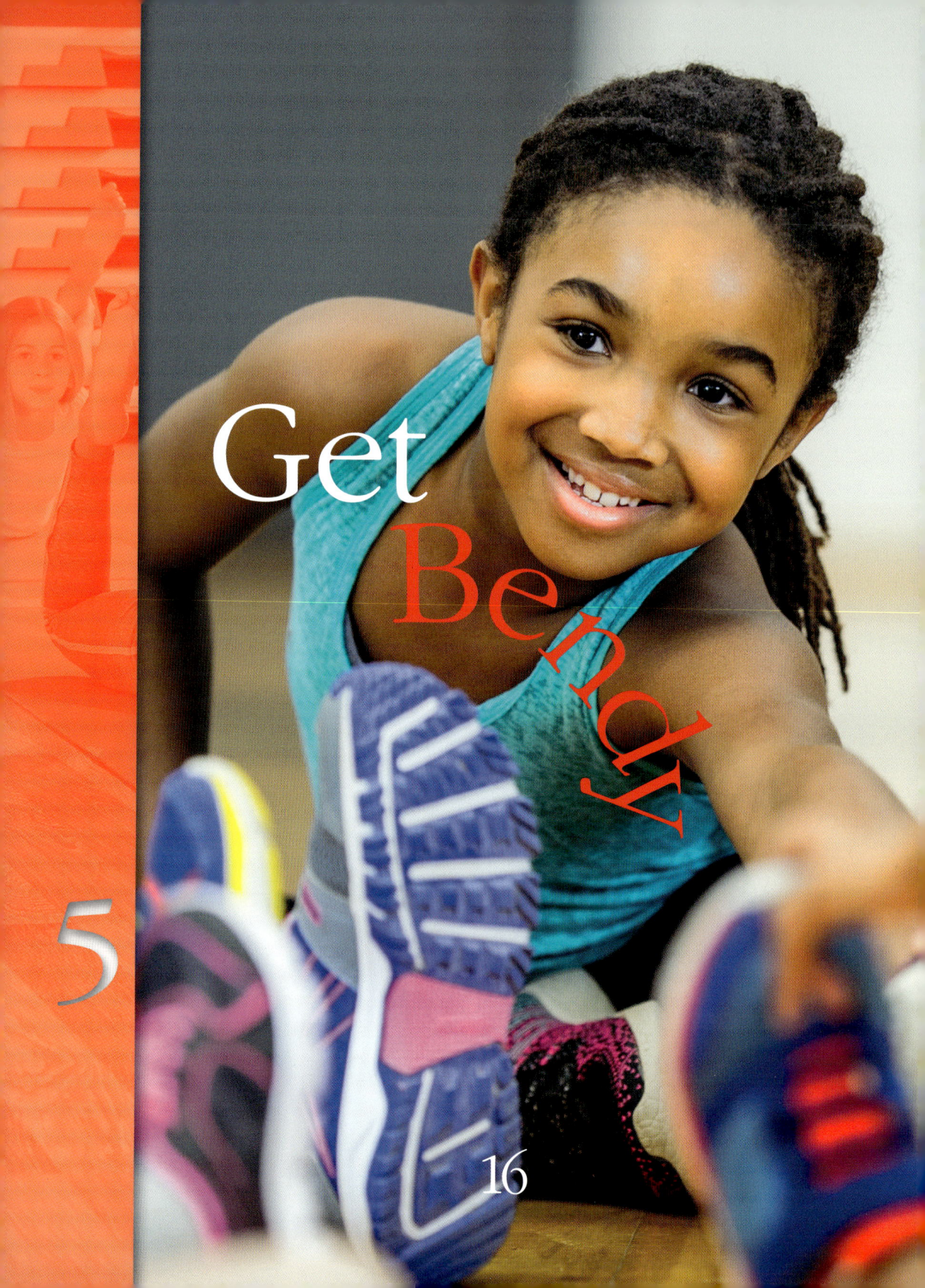

Get Bendy

5

16

Stretch gently before you run or play sports. Then stretch again after. Stretching helps blood flow into your muscles. It loosens them up and makes you more flexible. Then you don't get hurt as easily.

Playing Twister is one fun way to stretch. Yoga is another. Yoga poses like cobra, cat, and downward-facing dog mimic how animals move. Or you can do toe-touches and side-stretches.

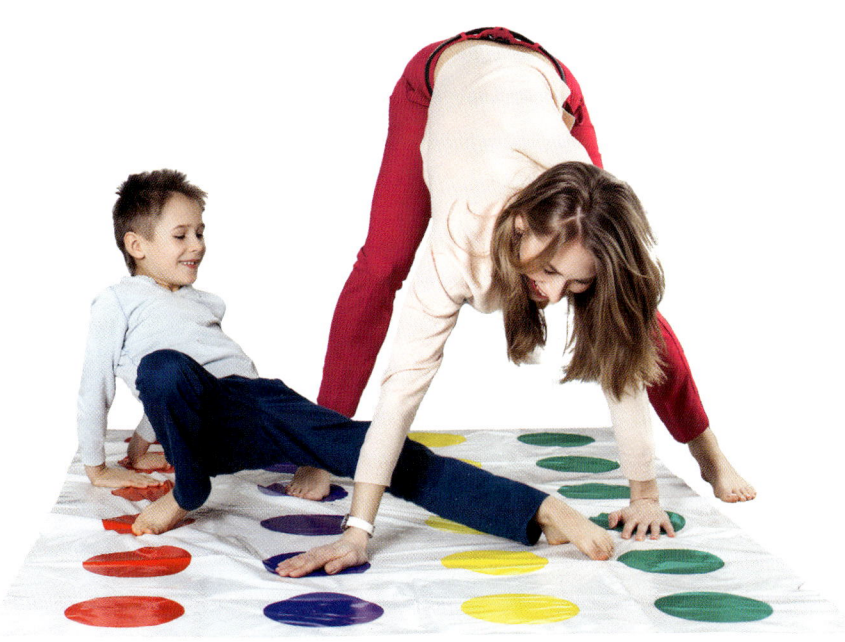

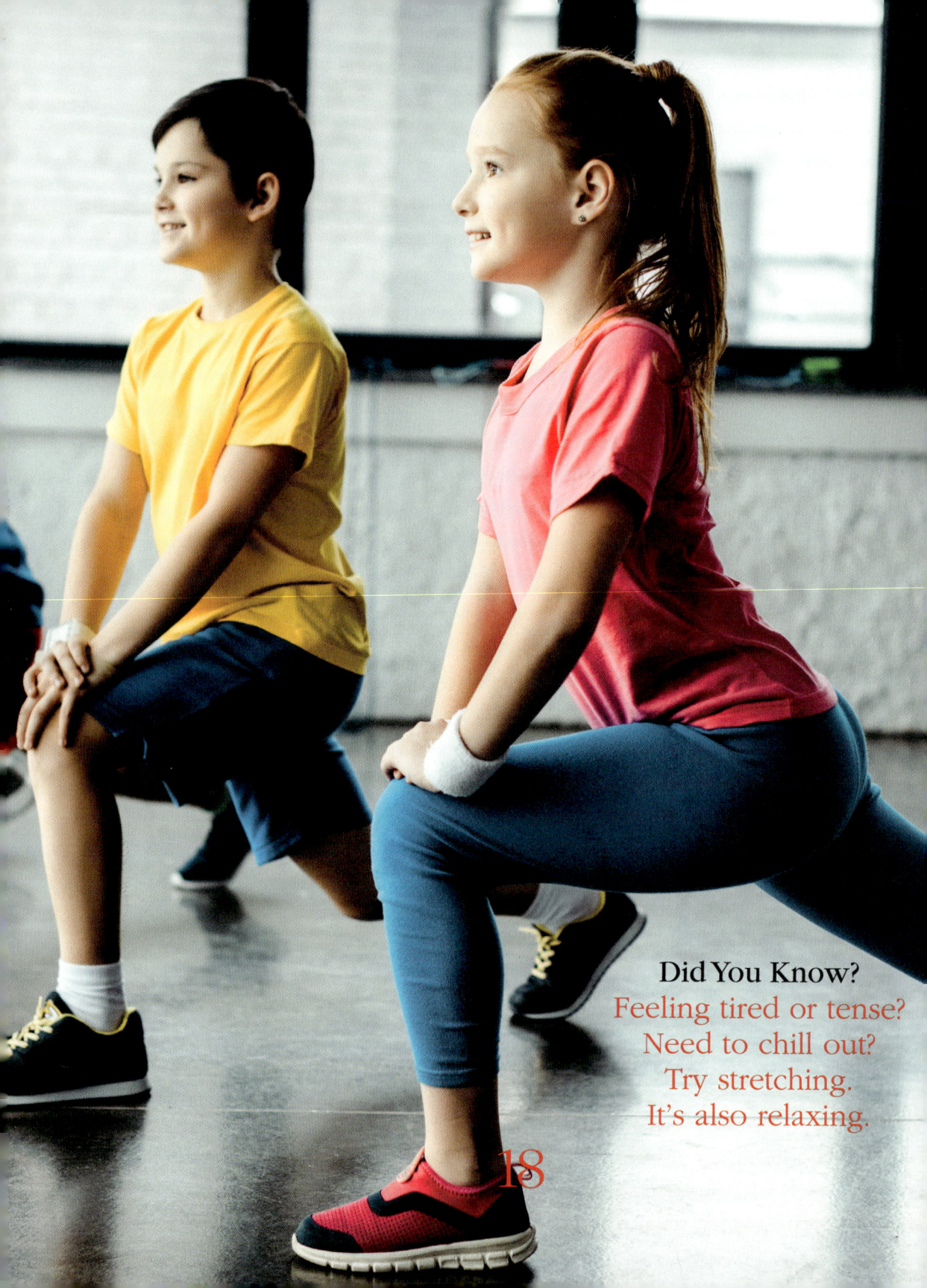

Did You Know?
Feeling tired or tense?
Need to chill out?
Try stretching.
It's also relaxing.

Have Fun with Fitness

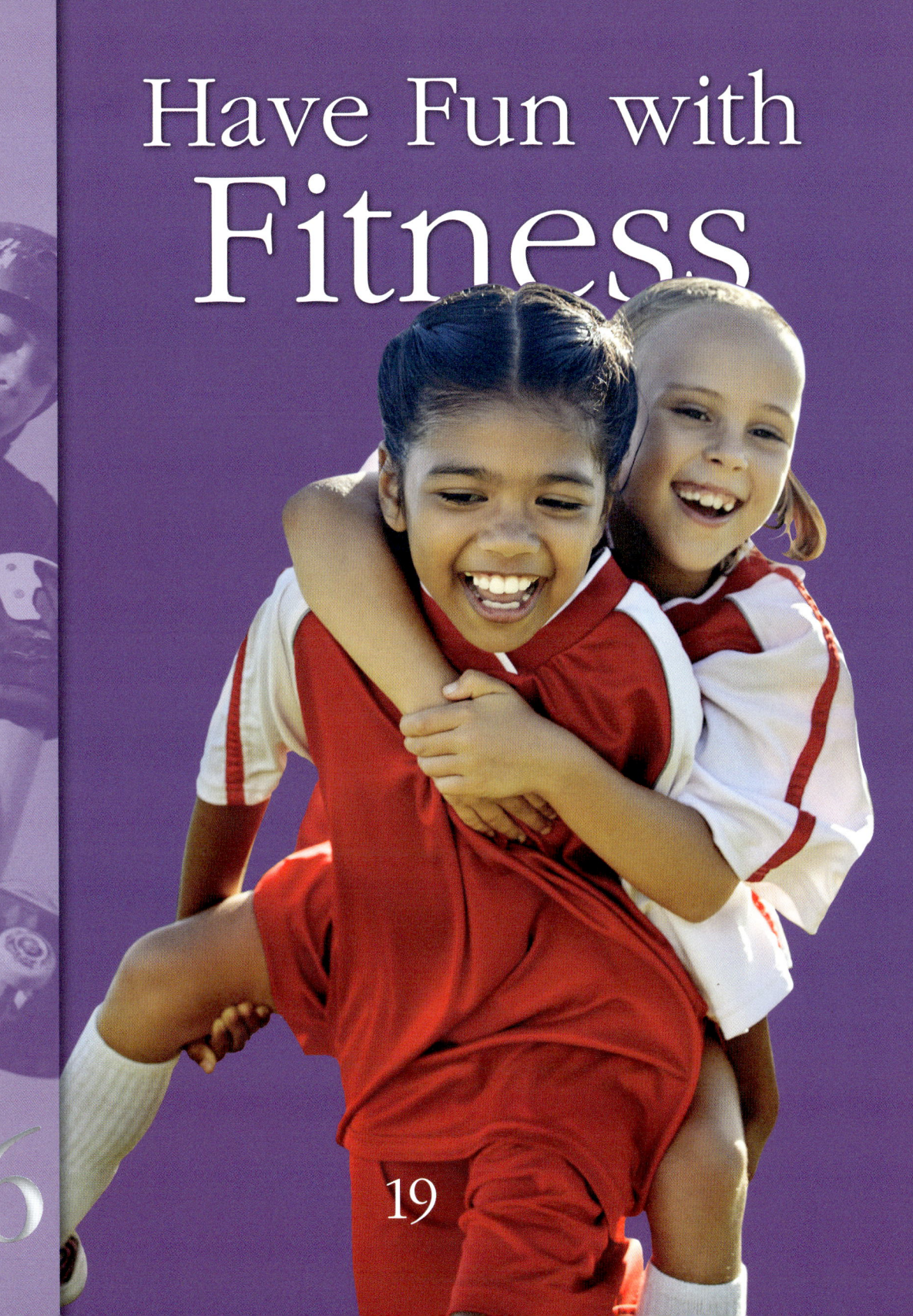

6

19

Your body is made to move. That's why you have more than 600 muscles! So, dance to your favorite music. Skip to school. Walk your dog. Being active can be fun. Join a game of hide-and-seek, tag, or tug-of-war.

Sports will keep you active as well. Play kickball or volleyball. Get on your bike or go for a swim. You can have fun with fitness every day. What will you do?

Think About It Is there a sport you'd like to play? Would you want to join a team?

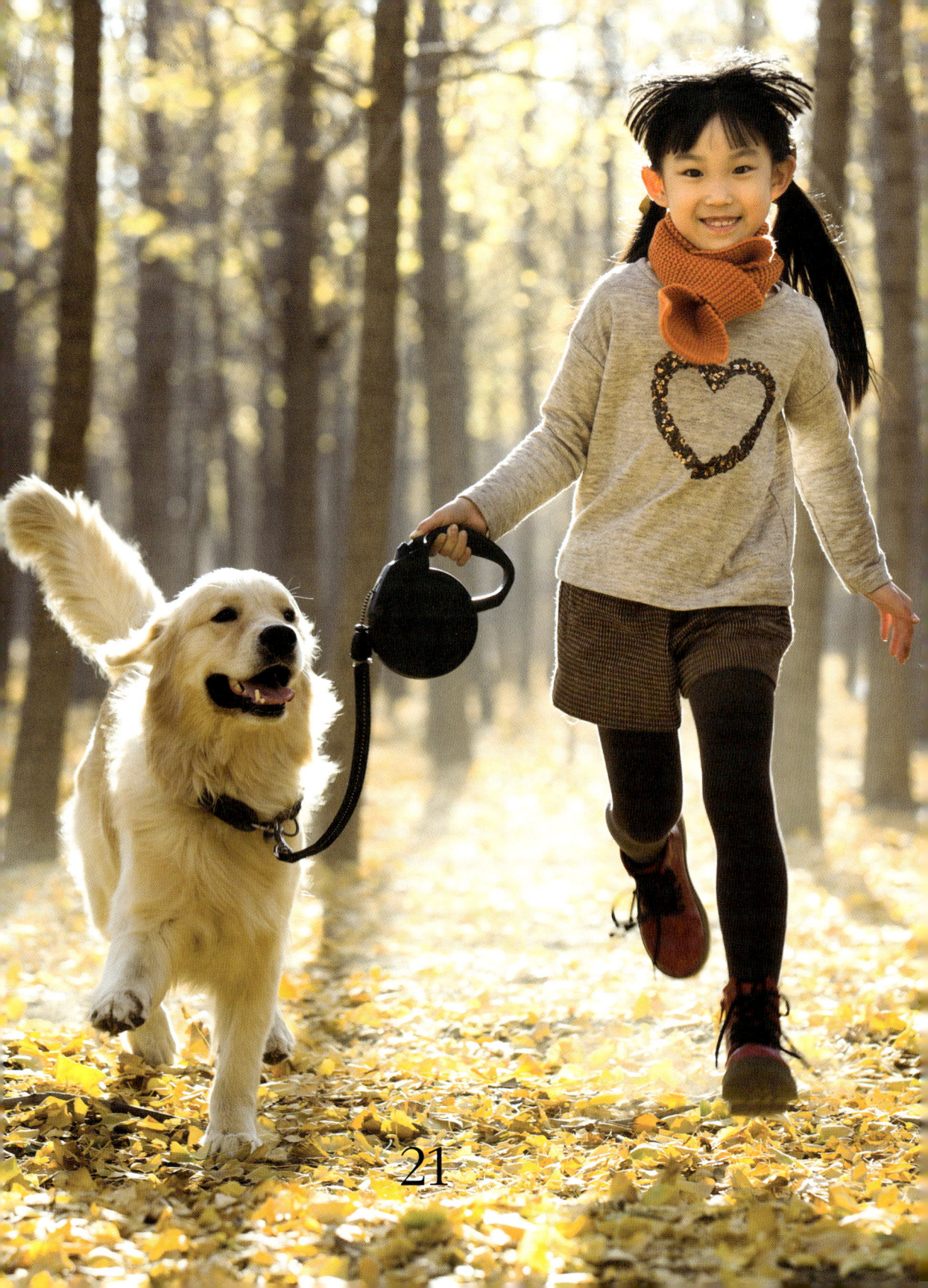

MORE TO EXPLORE
FANTASTIC FACTS

Experts say kids should do muscle-building activities at least three times a week.

The heart is the strongest muscle in the body.

Swimming is a great way to be active. It's good for your heart AND your muscles.

Active children are more likely to be active adults.

Playing sports can boost your self-confidence.

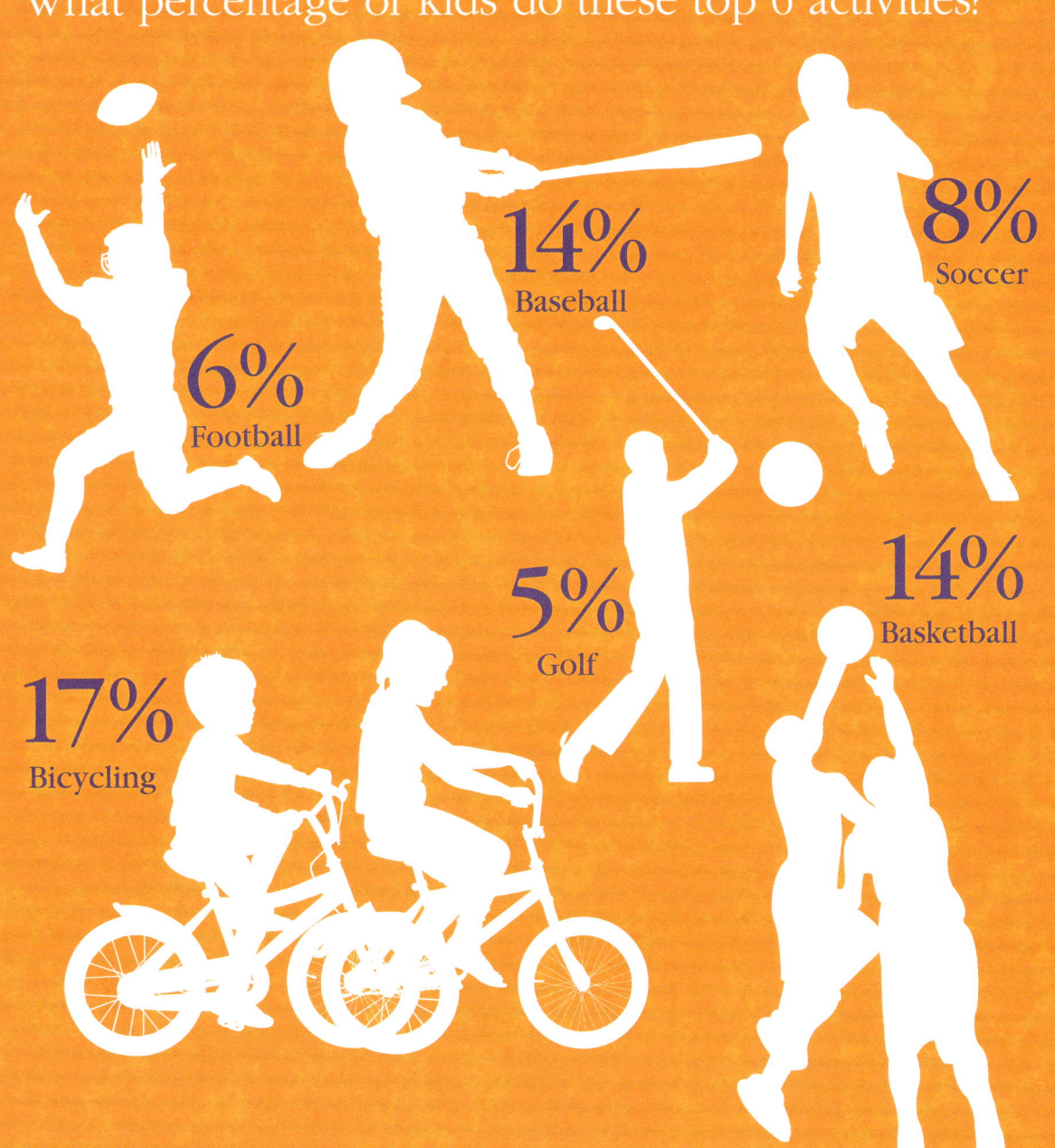

MORE TO EXPLORE
RESOURCES

Glossary

concentrate (KAHN-sun-trayt) To focus attention on one thing or activity.

core muscles (KOHR MUHS-uhls) The muscles deep within your stomach and back that support your spine and pelvis.

endurance (en-DUR-enss) The ability to do something physically or mentally demanding for a long time.

flexible (FLEK-suh-buhl) Able to bend easily.

mimic (MIHM-ik) To copy or imitate.

performance (per-FOR-muhns) The act of doing something, like a task or a sport.

puberty (PYOO-ber-tee) The time when a child's body changes into an adult's body.

Read More

Chang, Kirsten. *Staying Active.* Minneapolis MN: Bellwether Media, 2022.

Finan, Catherine C. *The Human Body.* Minneapolis MN: Bearport Publishing Company, 2021.

Index

brains, 8
energy, 5, 8
fitness, 20
flexibility, 5, 17
heart, 14, 22
muscles, 11, 12, 14, 20, 22
sleeping, 8
sports, 11, 12, 17, 20, 22, 23
stretching, 17, 18
sweating, 14
yoga, 17

TOP RANK is published by Black Rabbit Books, P.O. Box 227, Mankato, MN, 56002. • COPYRIGHT © 2025 Black Rabbit Books. All rights reserved. No part of this book may be reproduced in any form without written permission from the publisher. • Top Rank is an imprint of Black Rabbit Books. • Edited by Alissa Thielges • Designed by Danny Nanos • Photographs © Getty: BJI/Blue Jean Images, 21, FatCamera 16–17, Image Source 12, Ryan McVay 6–7; Shutterstock: adike, 20, altanaka, 2–3, Croisy, 14 (bkgd), Fotokostic, 11, Gregory Johnston, 15, LightField Studios, 8–9, 18, Monkey Business Images, cover, 1, 4, NadzeyaShanchuk, 5, Olena Chukhil, 17, PeopleImages.com – Yuri, A, 19, Pressmaster, 13, Save nature and wildlife, 23, Sergey Novikov, 10–11, Shot4Sell, 14 • Printed in the United States of America

Library of Congress Cataloging-in-Publication Data: Names: Snow, Peggy, author. | Title: Active and fit / by Peggy Snow. | Description: Mankato, MN: Black Rabbit Books, [2025] | Series: Top rank: healthy and happy | Ages 8–11 | Grades 4–6 | Identifiers: LCCN 2023058206 | ISBN 9781632357939 (library binding) | | ISBN 9781645820710 (ebook) | Subjects: LCSH: Children—Health and hygiene—Juvenile literature. | Physical fitness—Juvenile literature. | Classification: LCC RJ101.7 .S56 2025 (print) | LCC RJ101.7 (ebook) | DDC 613.7/042—dc23/eng/20240118 | LC record available at https://lccn.loc.gov/2023058206